Mastering Your Type 2 Diabetes and Heart Disease

By: Maggie Masters

Table of Contents

Introduction 1

Chapter 1 7

Why Are We Killing Ourselves? 7

Chapter 2 23

"Where's the Beef?" © 23

Chapter 3 44

The Two Largest Killers of Baby Boomers 44

Chapter 4 68

Storytime: A Type 2 Diabetes Story 68

Chapter 5 74

Storytime: A Heart Disease Story 74

Chapter 6 79

Covid 19 and the Added Risk 79

Chapter 7 88

Covid and the Cost of Healthcare in Retirement 88

Chapter 8 93

Baby Boomers - We are the World - 93

Chapter 9 99

My Final Thoughts 99

References 101

Introduction

"One day you turn around, and it's summer

Next day you turn around, and it's fall

And the springs and the winters of a lifetime

Whatever happened to them all."©

- composed by Jimmy Van Heusen, written by Sammy Cahn.

Let's face it! The retirement dream for millions of Baby Boomers has been tainted by illness, concerns about Medicare, and the health care system. The emergence of Covid 19 in the past few years only added tragic devastation to those deep concerns that we already had. It is projected that out of the approximate 80 million Baby Boomers today almost 65 million will get Covid and almost 2 million will die.

Those are scary numbers, but they pale in comparison to the dangers posed by Type 2 Diabetes and heart disease. This is because 25% of all Boomers will have Type 2 Diabetes and 70% will have some form of heart disease. 70%!! Let's face it 70% is a terrible number! This means that of the over eighty million Boomers alive today, over fifty five million will have heart disease. Think about that. Just think about that number. Over fifty five million Boomers with some form of heart disease. Did this information have anything to do with the surge in Baby Boomer retirement since the start of Covid 19?

As if life for retiring Baby Boomers with heart disease or diabetes don't have enough to deal with, Covid has changed everything. The requirements for general healthcare, long term care, rehabilitation care and others have changed in many ways. After more than a year of allowing no visitors, struggling with spread in closed facilities such as nursing homes and rehab centers, the industry is snake bitten.

A crisis in healthcare in the United States was on the horizon before the first drops of covid were found. With an onslaught of retiring Baby Boomers looking to Medicare and Medicaid for coverage, the system will be strained.

Before Covid many places in the healthcare system were already feeling the effects of an aging Baby Boomer generation. There was a shortage of professionals trained to care for an ever increasing aged population. As Boomers age they need more support from hospitals, urgent care centers, nursing homes and the growth of diversified living centers. Independent living, Assisted Living, Memory Care and Skilled Nursing Care began to merge in urban areas into large living spaces for the elderly. With this growth comes a shortage of doctors, nurses, dieticians, physical therapists, cardiologists, endocrinologists, and neurologists. There is even a shortage of billing clerks and massage therapists. Today healthcare is one of the fastest growing career opportunities in America. This is exasperated by the aging of the professionals working in this field. There are more nurses over age fifty in America today than those under 50.

We are about to see a health care system stripped bare by Covid and experiencing severe shortcuts as never before. Your healthcare – our healthcare will depend not only on less people but on many years less experience. This is the reason you get so many pushing the government to help in this situation. But is the answer in larger urban care centers or smaller local centers where Baby Boomers live and work today.

The Affordable Care Act of 2009 is geared to community care but leaves a gap in acute care. We need both. Boomers will be using local care centers, but we will certainly need acute care as well. That is unless we change our lifestyles to prevent heart disease and Type 2 diabetes. Alternative medicine and homeopathic remedies might be available as well.

Type 2 Diabetes is absolutely a lifestyle disease, and its worst effects can be avoided with lifestyle changes. On the other hand, the risk of heart disease increases with age and lifestyle. The complications of Covid 19 also increase with age. Having diabetes or heart disease could make a bout with Covid deadly when it didn't have to be. These conditions make catching Covid a much greater risk.

This it is complicated by the fact that Boomers don't feel our age. Don't tell us we are elderly! We feel we are in the prime of our lives. It was shocking to hear we were at higher risk for Covid because we were "older".

This little guide will help all baby boomers, and hopefully, those who come after us to plan a retirement that is the best life possible.

This means having the healthiest retirement possible. To do that, I will look at these two major diseases – heart disease and Type 2 Diabetes. What causes them? Can they be reversed? We know they can be prevented in many cases but what about the inherited cases? What can we do about that? What are the signs and symptoms of these diseases and what can you do if you develop those symptoms?

Both diseases can be silent – which means they can do a lot of damage before they show any outward symptoms. A healthier lifestyle is the answer to their stealthiness. Without a doubt at least 60% of all Baby Boomers have some sort of serious health issues. This includes arthritis and hypertension in addition to diabetes and heart disease. There will be a lot of need for doctors with geriatric experience, dieticians for aging bodies and a deep dive into all the types of medications Boomers take.

In addition to the basic facts, I will also be sharing with you some stories from Boomers who suffer from Type 2 Diabetes and heart disease. These are tough, emotional stories with truth about the challenges these diseases cause. But this wouldn't be a "Let's face it! Maggie Masters book' if it didn't include hope. I will offer you hope. You can beat the odds and YOU can have a great, healthy aging process. A retirement of fun, friends, family, travel, play, volunteer work, continued growth, and education is still possible for all. We just have to make the moves to make it happen.

So, I will start out by looking at the lifestyles of Americans and how our health is impacted by them. We are what we eat. Believe it. This is followed by an overview of each of these two diseases. Then comes Storytime. Hold onto your hat! These are intense stories. This will bring us back to Covid and its impact on patients with these diseases. What about "Long Covid"? How does it impact those of us with diabetes and/or heart disease?

When it comes to aging with these medical conditions there are always questions about resources and finances. How has Covid 19 affected the healthcare system of 2022? What's different now and how do we handle those differences? Along with this I'll take another look at what it costs for healthcare in our later years. What are the possible costs specifically for these two diseases?

Then it's Storytime again but these stories are filled with hope. I promised you hope and here it is. Stories of living and thriving with diabetes and heart disease. Stories to bring hope. Then continuing with hope, I'll look at what we, the Baby Boom generation, have learned from our experiences with Covid and these diseases. We have always set the pace and right or wrong paved the road for future generations. Hopefully we can do so again, with positive health outcomes and less disease in future generations.

After all we are Baby Boomers – "We are the world!" Just don't blink.

"Next thing you know your better half of fifty years is there in bed

And you are praying God takes you instead

Trust me friend a hundred years

Goes faster than you think, so don't blink"©

- Kenny Chesney

Chapter 1

Why Are We Killing Ourselves?

The American Lifestyle

Here in the United States, we pride ourselves on our lifestyle. We believe we have the best way of life in the world. We are the freest. We are the most affluent. We are the most successful. Let's face it, we are also some of the unhealthiest people in the entire world. We excel at overeating and lack of exercise. As my mother always said, we are "digging our graves with a spoon."

This is because 25% of all Boomers will have Type 2 Diabetes and 70% will have some form of heart disease. 70%!! Let's face it 70% is a terrible number! This means that of the over eighty million Boomers alive today, over fifty-five million will have heart disease. Think about that. Just think about that number. Over fifty-five million Boomers with some form of heart disease.

In the pandemic year and the years ahead of us, the Baby Boomers are entering an age when their health is more at risk than ever before. We are much more susceptible to senility, Alzheimer's, dementia, brittle bones and weakened immune systems. Add to that natural aging process, the abusive lifestyles so many of us have lived for so long. This situation will lead to a healthcare system that was questionable in terms of handling the load before Covid. That system is on life support itself in many places.

Thus, healthcare is one of the fastest growing fields of industry in the country. The current demand already exceeds the supply by about ten percent. Even as we have remained the most affluent country in the world, our life expectancy has fallen behind other affluent nations. Now it is in decline. Mortality rates among the working adults in lower socioeconomic classes have dropped slowly over the past forty years. Before the pandemic, the life expectancy of the average American was 78 years while other developed countries stood at 83 years old. This difference could be blamed on many factors including the lack of universal health care, lower education levels, public health crisis, poor federal drug   oversight, the deindustrialization of the American economy and last but not least, unhealthy lifestyle.

It is these unhealthy lifestyles that lead Baby Boomers into the two major diseases I wish to discuss in this book. These unhealthy lifestyles include obesity, smoking, and lack of exercise, drug use, and alcohol use. The most preventable of these is cigarette smoking leading to half a million deaths per year. Many Baby Boomers have given up smoking only to watch their grandchildren puff away. Many of us began smoking before we really knew how deadly it was. Once we did know, we were left with an addiction as bad as an illicit drug to overcome. Kudos to so many Baby Boomers for finally overcoming it.

A major cultural culprit for Baby Boomers is the fast food we all grew up on. The percentage of obese Americans skyrocketed from 1999 to 2018 increasing by 11%. By 2018, 42% of Americans fell into the category of obese. At the same time 4% of the population went from obese to morbidly obese. Food is not the only factor in obesity as a lack of exercise and consumption of alcohol are major contributors.

When it comes to the healthiest nation in the world, that honor goes to Singapore. Italy and Australia follow close behind. The United States on the other hand is the 33rd healthiest nation in the world. Very few Americans can count their lifestyles as healthy. This puts Baby Boomers in a precarious situation as we age. An unhealthy lifestyle leaves us vulnerable to Type 2 Diabetes and chronic or acute heart disease.

If you have a healthy lifestyle which includes eating right, exercising in moderation, avoiding as much stress as possible, and staying away from alcohol, drugs, and tobacco you can prevent many of the diseases of old age. Unfortunately, too many of us do not have healthy lifestyles and as we age, we are susceptible to heart disease, diabetes, arthritis, and more.

Although medicine has improved a lot in our lifetime, so have unhealthy lifestyles. Studies done among Boomers from 1988 to 1994 showed that overall health was lower than previously thought. More than half of all Boomers get no regular exercise at all. We do drink more water than our predecessors, usually in all the cups of coffee we consume.

Can we say our lives have been more stressful than our parents? Not likely as they faced the Great Depression, the specter of Hitler and the Nazis and World War Two. However, we have created a lifestyle of immense stress through its drive for success and conspicuous consumerism. There have never been enough hours in the day for us and there has never been enough success to satisfy us. We are a generation of "never enough."

All this stress, smoking, obesity, lack of exercise and unhealthy eating is leading us into a retirement plagued by heart disease and type two diabetes. With that will come the rising costs of medical care, prescription drugs, the portions of our medical bills not paid by Medicare, Medicaid or insurance and the cost of long-term care? Talk about stress! Uncovered long term care alone will cost upwards of $50,000, do you have $50,000 set aside for you and your spouse? What if prescription drugs cost tens of thousands of dollars over the remainder of your life?

In the United States these financial burdens are on us. In another country you might have a government or social program covering these things. But in the U.S., you are paying for your lifestyle mistakes yourself even though your lifestyle was in complete compliance with the larger culture.

McDonalds and Burger King are not going to pay for your heart disease. Over 40% of Boomers are obese compared with 29% of our parents. This just might be the biggest lifestyle issue for Boomers, and I will dedicate the next chapter to its origins and viable solutions. It is easy to see that we were the first generation to grow up with fast food and workplaces where we sat at a desk in front of a machine all day.

According to a leading researcher in the field ""Obesity has implications for increased diabetes risk, hypertension, and high cholesterol, among other health issues." The same report showed a remarkable increase in hypertension, high cholesterol, and diabetes along with obesity.

We will deal with arthritis and autoimmune diseases in a future book but understand that obesity is a partial reason for all those canes, walkers and scooters Baby Boomers take everywhere with them.

Mobility and balance are far greater issues for us than they were for our parents and their parents. My grandmother passed at age 85 and she was still living alone and doing everything for herself. I never remember hearing her complain of arthritis or chronic pain. Let's face it! I complain of chronic pain at least ten times a day and I am almost 20 years younger than my grandmother was when she died.

What can you do about all this now? Well first we will look at and understand this lifestyle – how did we get here and what can we do about it? Since food and obesity is a huge factor in this lifestyle and since we are the first generation to live with fast food daily, I will take a deep dive into this topic in chapter two. In the meantime, I will take a little more time in this chapter to look at the other two major lifestyle factors impacting the Baby Boom generation: stress and sedentary lifestyles.

Stress in our Lives

There are and have been many causes of stress in the lives of Baby Boomers. Whether you are already retired or still working, you have or do experience these many causes of stress. The top causes include work stress for those not yet retired. Health issues stress all of us as do many financial stresses. If you are or were a caregiver there is a special stress associated with this role. Of course, we have all been stressed by the many aspects of the Covid 19 pandemic. Personal safety, politics, and personal relationships are also often a cause of stress.

It is still not well known how stress functions in respect to our health. Are there different stressors, distribution of stressors, stress effects and stress mediators between generations? Are Boomers more susceptible than other generations? If so, why? What are the specific stressors facing the Baby Boom generation? Many studies have been or are currently being conducted on these questions.

This research is carried out via a survey or questionnaire given to various groups of Baby Boomers. Each Boomer is asked to give a rating to their level of stress and anxiousness in five of the areas mentioned above. These five areas included safety, politics, health, relationships, and finances.

From these studies comes something called the National Anxiety Score – this one for the Baby Boom generation specifically. The mean scores are 0-100 and the score for 2018 was 51 – a seven-point increase from the previous year.

The greatest anxiety was around finances in 2018. However, by 2022 these changes for Baby Boomers to anxiety over health and the healthcare system.

A few other findings that were significant included:

> There is more concern about health and finances than politics and relationships.

People of color are more stressed than Caucasians,

People on Medicare and/or Medicaid are more likely to be anxious than those who still have private insurance.

Those taking the survey also mostly agreed that one's mental health affects one's physical health. 75 percent of respondents felt that poor mental health was a negative drag on the economy and half felt there was a mental health stigma in the country that prevented some people from getting help. 1000 Baby Boomers participated in this study. The study shows that stress increases every year as the Boomers age.

Physicians have stated for many years that stress can bring on headaches, chest pain, changes in appetite, sleep issues, chronic pain, insomnia, stomach issues, fatigue, difficulty concentrating and muscle tension. This is only a sampling of the daily health consequences of stress. Long term consequences can include type two diabetes and heart disease. Stress weakens the immune system and makes us more vulnerable to colds, flu, and of course Covid 19.

So how can we Baby Boomers reduce the stress in our lives? There are many avenues and roads for dealing with stress, the first of which is to acknowledge it. Find out what triggers your stress. Just remember that stress is a normal aspect of life and cannot be completely avoided. It can however be tempered and treated so that it does not have a negative impact on your health.

Taking care of yourself in the face of stress requires that you acknowledge the stress and that you know what triggers stress for you. Another thing to know and remember is that what is stressful for you might not be stressful for someone else. Everyone has different things that trigger their stress. How does your body feel when you are in stress? Does your stress show up in your muscles, your stomach, and your head? The more you know about your stress the easier it is to dissipate or manage it.

If you want to prevent your stress reaction all together a deep understanding of its cause, your triggers, your response and how your body acts it out. It is better to prevent stress than to attempt to mitigate it. Perhaps you can prevent it with better sleep, better health, exercise, vitamins, or other practices. These types of activities can prevent stress from impacting your health and your life. By responding appropriately to your own stress signals or catching it before it is out of control, you can prevent many of these negative stress responses.

If you want good health in retirement or leading up to it, it is vital to control your stress. While you may be faced with stressors such as loneliness and loss of independence. You might be bored, experience your friends passing away and a less than satisfactory social life. This leads to increased blood sugar, changes in your metabolism, higher blood pressure and increased cortisol.

Heart disease and diabetes, upset stomach, dementia, depression, and obesity are the results of all this stress. Inflammation levels in the body are increased by stress leading to heartburn and heart disease. High cholesterol and high blood pressure increase chances of heart disease. This same inflammation can cause vascular dementia. Chronic stress impacts your metabolism and can lead to obesity. These metabolic changes can cause the flight or fight response and lead to deadly diabetes. Depression is also a result of stress.

Sedentary Lifestyle

Aside from smoking which I addressed briefly earlier; the other major culprit is the lack of exercise in our very sedentary lifestyles. As you will see in the next chapter there are major repercussions for being the first generation in history to live off of fast food. Let's face it there are just as major repercussions for being the first generation in history to have a computer as one of their primary work tools. This computer has tied to many people to their desk for the entire workday. This leaves us with the need for exercise before or after the workday.

Now think of all the stresses we just discussed and how much time do Boomers have for exercise around balancing work and family. That has been a definite challenge for Boomers throughout their careers. Our sedentary lifestyle paired with fast food has led to extremely high levels of obesity, diabetes, and heart disease. It's a vicious cycle. Physical inactivity, overwork, smoking and obesity with stress lead us into chronic illness. Then the stress of chronic illness just adds to the overeating and lack of physical exercise. Both genetic and behavioral factors work against Boomers having a healthier lifestyle.

Studies show that most Americans have exceptionally low levels of physical activity. At the same time over ten million of us are taking care of our own aging parents. We know that caregivers have even less time for taking care of themselves or exercising. On top of this lack of exercise, these caregivers only add more stress – the stress of being a caregiver. It is a vicious circle as studies show the more stress the less physical activity. The less physical activity, the more stress. Add to that the smoking and stress induced eating and you have a pretty lousy lifestyle.

U.S. government studies looked for signs of poor health such as smoking, diet, sedentary lifestyles, and thoughts. Findings concluded that caregivers were more likely to have these negative behaviors and more women than men. Even if you are not a caregiver, this sedentary lifestyle can creep in and rob you of your life. It is particularly disturbing to see the statistics on how much sitting retired Baby Boomers do.

Most of us think of retirement as a time when we will be free of stress and ready to do all those things on our wish list. Few of us think of retirement as a time when we just sit around most of the time doing nothing. Now be realistic and face it, we spend an awful lot of time sitting around. You might be reading a novel. You might be finishing a short walk around your house. You might be engrossed in something on your television or listening to a podcast. With any of these activities there is either very little or no physical activity. You could be sitting all day.

It sounds great! It sounds relaxing and it sure sounds like retirement. However, sitting too much, too long, is hazardous to your health. You might think you remember sitting all day at the office too, but you didn't. You got up for coffee, for breaks, to deliver materials or reports. You walked to meetings, to the cafeteria and you lost your way.

There is plenty of unnoticed walking in the workplace. And there is plenty of unnoticed sitting in the home front. On average we increase the amount of time we sit by 4 and ½ to six hours a day from about 3 - 4 hours before retirement. Sitting for a long time in blocks of time is certainly detrimental to your health. You use fewer active muscles in retirement unless you are incredibly active.

Loss of mobility, balance, and even mortality can come from sitting too much. Excessive sitting can lead to Type 2 diabetes, cancer, increases in cholesterol and high blood pressure. These things can lead to strokes, heart disease, obesity, even cancer. Let's face it, these are only some of the diseases we can get from too much sitting.

It will take you an hour or an hour and fifteen minutes to counteract your daily sitting. It also can't hurt to limit the amount of time you sit without walking around. So set a timer and take a walk around your house every half hour. If you are engrossed in watching a television show, walk around the room during commercials. Don't sit down to have a phone conversation. Walk around. Walk around any chance you get. Do away with the sedentary lifestyle.

Remember over 50% of Boomers self-report a sedentary lifestyle. This lifestyle is suicidal so get up and do something. If your lifestyle does not include physical activity on a daily routine basis, then you are not as healthy as you think. Live a sedentary life and open yourself up to all the chronic illnesses that Boomers are prone to and face disabilities much earlier in life.

Fewer Boomers are still smoking and dying of emphysema than their parents did but more of us have heart disease from high cholesterol and high blood pressure. Ask around your senior apartment complex. You will think everyone is on blood pressure medications because the response will be so overwhelming. If you are living a sedentary lifestyle, then you are burning less calories and are ripe for becoming overweight. You are not using your muscles enough so they are not as strong as they could be. You might have problems with your immune system or have weaker bones. These are just a few consequences of a sedentary life.

My Conclusions

That gives you a better idea of the kinds of stress and non-activity that has characterized the lifestyles of Baby Boomers. In the next chapter I will delve deeply into the issue of obesity and the "fast food generation." Let's face it – we were at one time in the last 50 years all into "where's the beef?"

That's the next chapter. In the meantime, try a little stress reduction.

Pray if it fits your life view.

Meditate even if you do not pray.

Exercise – go swimming.

Take a yoga class.

Take the time to practice mindfulness.

Join or form a support group dealing with everyday stress.

Be active – take your mind off the negative – volunteer.

Now let's move on and take a deep dive into our sedentary fast-food lifestyles. Let's find out why we are killing ourselves.

My Fast Food

"Bloated, salty, and greasy,

My body does not like thee,

Yet I devour you

And inch along to heart attack.

I have to have you,

My certain death.

I must possess you:

Cheap fix; expensive consequences.

I would consume you every day,

Every meal,

And still not have my fill–

With disastrous results.

Packaged simply,

A benign answer

To my problems.

But you only create them.

You go down easy,

But upset my system soon after.

I can't sleep, can't think, can't eat–

Can't live.

Fast, fried, and flirty,

Desirable and disgusting,

Tasty and tasteless–

My oxymoron.

I must resist.

I must cease and desist.

But I don't want to.

So, I line up for you again,

And again.

And again." ©

- April 9, 2018, by Carrie @ poet in the pantry-

Chapter 2

"Where's the Beef?" ©

American Fast Food - "Two all Beef Patties, Special Sauce, Lettuce, Cheese, Pickles, Onions on a Sesame Seed Bun"

A generation of "Boomers" is moving into retirement in the same way that they moved into changing the world in the 1960s. As they do so they are reclaiming their place in pop culture, but many are moving away from a staple of that culture. That staple is fast food.

Baby Boomers were the first generation to experience life from the perspective of a consumer. They grew up on television, developed the computer age and 24-hour news on cable. Rock and roll was born and fueled by mass audiences for the first time in history. Now as they move into a period of life without the worries of raising a family or running a business. Boomers belong to themselves again and they turn again to influencing popular culture, what we eat, what we do, who we listen to.

Now the concerns are health care, quality of life, financial establishment and more. Right in the middle of this is our addiction to fast food and our desire for a healthier lifestyle. We are or hope to be more active than our parents and their parents. Suddenly marketers are paying attention to seniors. This has never been the case before. With this power perhaps this generation can have an impact on not only what they eat, but what everyone eats.

Let's face it, in America we love our burgers and fries. We love our "fast food." The problem is it doesn't really love us back as it attacks our waistline and our health. "You are what you eat," they say. If that's true than many Americans are hamburgers and fries.

As stated in the previous chapter, it's time to take a deep dive into the American way of eating and its impact on our health. As I said before, Boomers are the first generation of Americans to always grow up with fast food available. First it was just burgers, fries, and a "coke." Or a shake. Then came Kentucky Fried Chicken and Pizza. Now there is every kind of food available in minutes on every street corner. Let's start by looking at the history of American Fast Food.

History of American Fast-Food Industry

Prior to 1950 Americans ate their meals at home or out of a lunchbox or brown bag at school and work. American fast food changed all that. It began in 1921 with the first White Castle but there was no real success until the 50's. Most people are familiar with the story of the McDonald brothers in 1948 and they were purchased by Ray Kroch. It was the genius of Ray Kroch and his ability to make fast food run like an assembly line that changed everything.

'White Castle was the country's first fast food chain when it opened in 1921 in Wichita, Kansas. White Castle was opened but did not see the success it would later have. It would take a bigger revolution in fast food to get White Castle rolling.

Just what exactly is "fast food"? It is usually defined as food that can be made and delivered in a very short period. This usually means it is precooked and frozen and just warmed on a grill or in a microwave. The first time the term became popular was in 1951 when it turned up in the Merriam-Webster dictionary for the first time.

Street vendors have been around since ancient times, but something new and different was born in the 1950s and blossomed in the 1960s into a cultural phenomenon. Fast food comes in many forms and types. In one part of the country a fast-food brand might offer different items than the same brand in another part of the country.

In the same year that Billy Ingram and Walter Anderson opened the first White Castle. A&W Root Beer created the first franchise activity. They offered their drink syrup to franchisees. It was in the 1930's when Howard Johnson offered the first restaurant franchise. Little did anyone know at this point how the concept of franchising would change the world of food in the United States?

McDonald's. Burger King, In-Out Burger, and Burger Chef

"Two All-Beef Patties, Special Sauce, Lettuce, Cheese, Pickles, Onions on a Sesame Seed Bun" ®

When the McDonalds brothers opened their first "fast food" restaurant in 1948, a new category of eating out was born. They were successful in this "walk up window" food service that was quick, hot, and delicious. Soon others began to follow in their footsteps. Burger King opened in the 1950s and Wendy's in 1969.

Non burger places like Taco Bell started in the 1950's while Kentucky Fried Chicken really got off the ground at the same time. Burgers and fries are the most popular type of fast food from the 1950s on. Beginning simply with burgers, fries and shakes these restaurants became household names in the 1960s even though most did not offer indoor sit-down eating. You could eat outside if there were tables, in your car or take your burgers home.

Soon burgers and fries were joined by chicken, onion rings, tacos, hot dogs, pizza, and ice cream. Dairy Queen, Burger King, KFC, Jack in the Box, and others grew up to challenge McDonald as Ray Kroc took over the brand. The simplicity of the offerings was part of the marketing in the 1960s as this Burger Chef jingle proclaimed...

"At Burger Chef

For a nickel and a dime, you'll get,

French fried potatoes

A big thick shake

And the greatest 15 cent hamburger yet." ©

Fast Food continued to grow and claim more and more of the restaurant market share. The American car culture of the 50s and 60s directly attributed to the growth of fast food. Drive-ins with car hops waiting on customers in their cars were popping up everywhere. A man named Troy Smith Sr. Bought a root beer stand in 1953 and converted it to a drive in. Soon the restaurant chain of SONIC was born and still exists as a drive in today.

A couple years later the most important event in the history of fast food took place as Ray Kroc began to franchise the McDonald's System. Within 4 years Kroc's McDonalds sold 100 million burgers. They were soon joined by Burger King, Burger Chef, Hardees and Wendys. Eventually Burger Chef was sold to Hardees and the brand died out.

Throughout the 50s and 60s there was a fast-food revolution well beyond burgers. We are all familiar with the tale of Colonel Sanders Kentucky Fried Chicken, but along came Dunkin' Donuts, Pizza Hut, Pizza King, Little Caesar,

Domino's, Arby's, Chick0fil-A, Taco Bell, and Subway. Today 80% of Americans still eat fast food at least once a month.

The founders of most of these fast-food chains grew up poor and were older when success finally came for them. They are the heart of the American Dream. Their franchises made success out of ordinary Americans who dared to dream, invest a few thousand dollars and a lot of sweat equity. The McDonald's brand of franchising opened up this brave new world to so many lower- and middle-class Americans.

So fast food was a hit – an enormous success – quintessentially American. "Supersize it!" ®. They said, Everyone knows the Big Mac jingle "Two All-Beef Patties, Special Sauce, Lettuce, Cheese, Pickles, Onions on a Sesame Seed Bun" ©. And I'm sure you also remember "You deserve a break today. So, get up and get away to McDonalds." ©

McDonalds was not only king of fast foods they were king of the fast-food jingle as well. All those catchy little ditties that stick in your head and play over and over. Here we are 20,30 years later and we still remember them. Are you loving it? Let's face it, "I'm loving it." ®

Because the fast-food industry is so large, every time someone wants to develop a new product or new packaging, new businesses must become involved. This is because the fast-food company is going to replicate that new product or new packaging hundreds of thousands of times for all its franchises all over the world. This is not true of all fast-food franchises. Some are not like McDonalds and don't require that every store have the same menu, the same products, and the same equipment. However most do and so the market for anything new is huge.

This makes fast food a more reactive than proactive industry. In the beginning it was all proactive but now it reacts to the changes and trends in the American economy. Instead of setting the trends, fast-food is usually following them instead. The innovation is coming from DoorDash, GrubHub, and Uber Eats. There was a push in the early 2000s to eat less fast-food and smaller portions, but it did not catch on. McDonalds will no longer "supersize it" but it's just as easy to order a larger fry than a medium one.

In a marketing ploy Kentucky Fried Chicken became KFC so that buyers would not be reminded that the chicken is fried. There is this emotional attachment to fast-food that makes it feel like a treat or a reward even if we eat it every day. Most customers are opposed to changing the recipes or making the food less salty and less fatty. Yet the companies are trying lower calories items such as salads, baked chicken, and the Impossible Burger.

Fast food is so big it is able to dictate to the suppliers and slaughter large amounts of animals according to the fast-food industry standards. When Dick and Mac McDonald ran their first restaurant, they offered over 25 different menus. Today's menus are much smaller and standardized.

The original McDonalds was a drive in with car hops. Closing this store, they developed their "Speedee Service System" assembly line. Cutting their menu also resulted in faster service. They then franchise the store and even before Ray Kroc enters the picture, the McDonald brothers have 8 restaurants.

Soon the franchise model was the future of fast-food including pizza and donuts. First there was Pizza Hut then Dominos offered delivery. Today's fast-food industry is really a matter of corporate giants owning multiple fast-food brands. Yum! Brands own Pizza Hut, KFC, Long John Silver's Taco Bell, and A&W.

The Impact of Fast-Food

It wasn't long before McDonald's controlled the supply chain for beef, pork, potatoes and even apples. Once breakfast started their influence spread to chicken farms as well. This led to large packing companies like IBP becoming the supplier of choice for hamburgers to the industry. McDonald's fish comes from Gorton's of Gloucester. KFC buys its chickens from Tyson, Perdue, and Pilgrim's Pride.

All of this led to big farms instead of family farms to produce standardized animal products. This has led to tremendous changes in agriculture and almost the end of family farms worldwide. It has also meant that most of the grain and corn grown worldwide is fed to animals instead of people.

As McDonalds was being born so were the Baby Boomers. We grew up on the Golden Arches. My kids loved Ronald McDonald, we saw him advertised everywhere, they memorized all those jingles. To us in the 60s we would walk miles across town to spend that precious change our Mom gave us on a shake with a burger and those awesome fries. It was well worth the walk, Oh how we loved McDonalds.

Wherever I traveled with my kids, large billboards declared "Food ahead" and they always begged to stop. Not only were they raised on the food produced by this industry, they were raised on its marketing as well. I admit I allowed it because it made my life easy and my waist line showed it.

At that time my generation had the cultural influence. We loved the newness of fast food and freedom from the kitchen. We were busy working parents and needed the break from feeding the kids unaware of the eventual consequences.

Of course, the major impact of fast food has been on the health and the waistline of Boomers. Even as Boomers try to make healthier and better food choices, the past echoes in both their minds and their stomachs. Giving up fast food is not so easy. Even as Boomers battle chronic illness fed by fast food, they still have a taste for it.

The impact of fast foods? Cancer, obesity, high cholesterol, high blood pressure, type 2 diabetes and more are rampant and chronic among Boomers. In the face of this Boomers are trying to create a much healthier American way of eating. It might still be fast and effortless like Door Dash or UberEats. But it might be healthier with salads and healthy entrees being delivered instead of fast food.

In addition, empty nesters are making more expensive, healthier food choices. The next question is what happens when they retire, and income becomes fixed or less available? Will this change the movement toward healthier foods? No matter what Baby Boomers do, we carry with us the consequences of fast food, processed foods, smoking and sedentary lifestyles. "You deserve a break today..." ®

Fast food products are designed to taste delicious be quick and easy to attain, and drive the hook deep into your psyche. Fast food companies and big agricultural interests are not interested in our health. If you can resist you can save money and improve your health.

Just take a look at the results of a survey done by the National Health and Nutrition Examination Survey known as NHANES. This survey taken with 46-year-old and 64-year-old looked at the intake of calories, sodium, fat, cholesterol, vegetables, fruits, water, vitamin C and fiber. Boomers' intake of calories, sodium, fat, and cholesterol was much higher than in previous generations. Vegetables, fruits, water, vitamin C and fiber intake were less. Thus, Boomers have taken in many more chronic disease related ingredients than their parents. Thus, we see record numbers of obesity, type 2 diabetes, and heart disease. It's the diet we have been eating all our lives that leads us here.

According to David Nico of *Diet Diagnosis* - "This is not a health crisis. This is a tragedy." Obesity is an insidious force in the quality of life for Boomers. It causes diabetes and heart disease as I have said. It also causes kidney failure and impacts every organ in the body. Obesity is the second leading cause of preventable deaths behind smoking.

Associate professor of community health at Ball State, in Indiana, Jagdish Khubchandani, names the cause of this obesity. "The dramatic rise in fast food culture in the Baby Boomer generation, fast life, increased consumption of processed food, more focus on medical care, and dwindling investments on education and preventive health.", according to Khubchandani are the cause of this obesity. "One could argue that Boomers came along at a time of great change in diet - more fast food. Activities have been engineered out of our lives - climbing stairs, doing household chores, TV remote controls. Boomers may be the age group that is most impacted."

It is not too late for us. We can change the way we eat, exercise and our attitudes. Yes, we have a higher risk for obesity, diabetes, and heart disease. Yes, we can change this. Dieting won't be enough. We must engage in cardio and strength building exercises. "The epidemic of obesity is the primary health concern for baby boomers. We were the first generation to grow up with fast food and computerized workplaces, which surely have had a hand in this," says Dr. Campagnolo. "Obesity has implications for increased diabetes risk, hypertension, and high cholesterol, among other health issues." "If you're obese, changing your diet is crucial to improving your health," says Dr. Campagnolo. It's not too late but those Big Macs, Whoppers and Extra-large pizzas have taken their toll. Let me share a story that will bring this point home even more.

Maggie's Story -Part One

The Way We Lived

I recently attended a Kenny Chesney concert, 60,000 fans strong and this one song seemed to sum up this chapter for me. See if you agree.

The body is a temple, that's what we're told

I've treated this one like and old Honky-Tonk

Greasy cheeseburgers and cheap cigarettes

One day they'll get me if they ain't got me yet.

I've been living in fast forward and now

I need to rewind real slow!

Famous lyrics from Kenny Chesney ©

"This was a real serious failure in our ability to choose good from bad and right from wrong." Our lifestyle choices were instant gratification while the devil was watching us and laughing. "Go ahead Maggie. Keep on killing yourself. Tamper with your body chemistry. Go ahead and lay the foundation for an early death, for a whole lot of medical turmoil ahead of you. We'll see who wins," says the devil. I really thought I was intelligent. I guess I wasn't thinking right. 65 years of dropping the curtain.

I am Maggie Masters, a not so unusual, perfectly common 71-year-old Baby Boomer, fighting to stay alive. I'm fighting to beat the odds not to die now that my years of hard work are behind me. 45 years of hard work to be exact. It took that long to retire, and I am not ready to die yet. Dammit! There is too much to do and too many adventures still left in me.

"Please Lord, I will be good. I know it's a bit late. Things will get better. I promise." Ouch! Hold on, where did this all come from? Are you reading this and nodding your head? Is it all too familiar?

I am writing this story for you. Perhaps together we can figure this out. How can we survive and continue on a good and happy path? Do you have Type 2 diabetes? Is it coupled with heart disease?

Well let's face it! We never thought twice when we took that first puff of a Marlboro Red or perhaps Kool menthol. We just did it. The more I kept trying to smoke those darn things, the more I coughed and the more addicted I became. I was only 14. By age 15 my bestie and I were running on our lunch hour, from school to her parents' house so we could smoke ourselves out. Lunch was 2 cigarettes and a bologna sandwich laced with too much yellow mustard.

True story my friend. Beth loved yellow mustard so much that her fingers and sweater sleeves always had yellow traces of lunch. I guess I will always remember her by this time in our lives. It was 1966.

I should have quit smoking when I was 16 and my mom had her first heart attack at age 47. She was driving me home from school when it hit. We had just turned down our street and I could tell she was in trouble. She clutched her chest. Instinctively I grabbed the wheel, put my foot over to the break and successfully stopped the car. I jumped out and ran the short distance to our house and got my dad. Our neighbors called the ambulance.

She lived thank God. My brother had died just 3 years earlier and I wasn't ready for her to go too. Sadly, her days of Camel Straights were not over. She had many more episodes, 14 altogether and at age 69 she finally had the big one. An aneurysm burst. When my step sisters cleaned out her closet, they found ten cartons of Camel Straights she had smuggled home from the Navy PX store in San Francisco.

My step dad knew she was a sneaky smoker. She would go into her bathroom, crack the window and puff away. Afterwards the tell-tale smell of that horrible air freshener spray drifts down the stairs and through the hallways. Oh Mom! Please stop! At the time, she was in her 50's

Mary Louise was a real beauty and a wonderfully talented homemaker, gardener, and artist. She was a devout Catholic and known as the Candy Lady at Sunday school. She always had a bag of candy in her purse for the kids at Church.

After they retired, my step-dad and she built a lovely house on the side of a hill overlooking Willits, a small northern California town – a lovely spot filled with gracious and kind neighbors. They lived in a trailer on the site pad for three years while building. Her health kept failing, and by the time they were ready to open the doors for her friends from the church for a party, she was in the hospital. Her peripheral artery disease had progressed, and walking was very hard.

She was a trim woman with a classy wardrobe. An entire wall of glass doors in their bedroom contained the beauty that was Mary Louise. After the funeral, the very next day,my stepsisters emptied the closets and took everything down the hill to St. Vincent's. My step father and I were devastated.Too much so to say stop .They realized when we all left it would be too hard for him to take on the task.

She was really gone! I sat in the guest room, huddled in a ball, and sobbed. Yet why did this not stop me from killing myself with cigarettes? I smoked until I was 55. 16 more years of killing myself – messing with my heart. Maggie, shame on you!

Now let's get back to talking about life threatening sin number two! Our American diet! First, I need to state that what I am writing here is not medical advice. This comes from my own experience after years of learning the hard way. I have done more than my share of reading, researching, and trying to figure it out. I've bought all kinds of remedies and wonder vitamins to save my life. I just couldn't quite make the curves before I fell off the cliff.

What's your story? I'd love to read it. You are welcome to share it with me at MaggieMastersAuthor@gmail.com.

Maggie's Story -Part Two

During my busy years as a young parent, I was trying to survive all the commotion that comes from living with an abusive alcoholic husband. I spent over 12 years allowing myself and my children to be abused. I wasn't concerned with my progressing heart disease and dietary consumption. I knew we had heart disease in our family, but eating was my medicine, my go to stress relief. Fats, beef, bacon, pork, sugar, donuts, and pies – I always had to work on my weight. My body was a roller coaster from one fad diet to another.

My energy levels were good, and I managed to silently keep killing myself. I was always trying to quit smoking – trying the next best aerobics or exercise class. I became a huge Richard Simmons fan. Yet it was all silently setting me up for failure. It was hereditary, genetic cholesterol overproduction mercilessly plugging up my arteries.

By age 40 I was testing way too high on the cholesterol meter, and I was put on statins- Crestor at first. What a nightmare! This wonder drug just nailed me – flat in bed sick! For over 20 years I went through 5 or 6 drugs - some worked, some didn't. All did cause leg cramps.

As dietary concerns piled up, I was put on one no fun diet after another. Success! I got off cigarettes and stayed off for 4 years. But in 1996, during a family medical emergency

I asked my stepson for a smoke. We were following the ambulance on an icy road in the early morning hours with my daughter in it. I asked, and he gave it to me! Hooked again! Hooked for 11 more critical years. I kept driving the nails into my own coffin.

I had my first heart catheter at age 47, with angina and high blood pressure as precursors. I was at normal body weight then, but I was still smoking. The next 18 years were just a process of piling on to the process of killing myself. I was smoking, drinking, and eating great steaks and seafood. I visited New Orleans a lot and enjoyed all the food that is a part of that lifestyle.

I had spent too many years trying to fix the heart disease and working with an older cardiologist who failed me. After he retired my new cardiologist gave me this important advice:

"Your cholesterol problem is genetic. It is in the food you are eating. Believe me it's in your family DNA. This causes your excess production of cholesterol. This cardiologist understood that I did not do well on statins and wisely put me on an injectable cholesterol medication – a pure miracle – no side effects! This change was made 7 years ago. I had already had bypass surgery. I recently had a heart catheter and after 7 years my arteries are clear and blockage free. Inflammation appears to be under control. Thanks to this smart young cardiologist I was able to do so.

When I was 62, my general practitioner told me I was pre-diabetic. What?? It was a shocker! What did that even mean? Within the next three years, I had a significant heart episode that went undiagnosed and untreated. I was very fatigued and had considerable shortness of breath.

I was still working and planning a three-week Alaskan cruise and overland adventure with my granddaughter. We were 2 months away from departure and out of an abundance of caution made an appointment with a longtime friend and doctor to check me out. Well old-time docs rock! They get to the bottom of things. He ordered a scan with contrast and looked at me and said, "Let's figure this out before your trip.

The results were shocking for me and my family. Within 4 days I had another heart cath. When I was coming out of anesthesiology, the operating room was quiet, very quiet – just a moment ago the staff had been playing music, laughing, and joking with me before they put me under.

Now after the procedure this silence – dead silence. They wouldn't tell me "Go home." Instead, they admitted me. By Monday morning I was having a triple bypass! The rest is history – However my heart and diabetic troubles were just beginning.

Then came the Covid 19 lockdown during which I developed full blown Type 2 diabetes. I had completely changed my entire diet, but heart disease and Type 2 diabetes go hand in hand. While caring for my grandsons during the lockdown, I gained 20 pounds. My grandsons and I were having a blast playing video games and eating great late-night snacks.

I became a great fan of this new way of fun, and I was eating my way to full blown Type 2 diabetes. I had wondered why my feet were getting so bad. I am still dealing with them. But now 7 years have passed since that surgery, and I have finally come up for air. I will not go into any more tales about my troubles as I don't want to scare you!

If I can say anything to give you inspiration – please put on the brakes with your diabetes, finding ways to heal. Diabetes is a devil in disguise. Heart disease isn't going away unless you get a new heart. Good luck on that one!

Let's talk!

 MaggieMastersAuthor@gmail.com.

Chapter 3

The Two Largest Killers of Baby Boomers

Type 2 Diabetes - What is it? What does it do?

Heart Disease - How many types are there? What does it do?

Type 2 Diabetes- What is it? What does it do?

As I mentioned in the introduction some 25% of all Baby Boomers will have Type 2 Diabetes. For the most part it is entirely related to lifestyle. Its worst effects can be avoided with lifestyle changes. It is projected that one in every four baby boomers will have type 2 diabetes. 1 in 4! Look around, is that you? Your spouse? Your brother? Your best friend? One in four. 25%.

There is more type 2 diabetes in the United States than in any other developed country. 25% have full blown diabetes and another 25% are pre diabetic. One out of every seven dollars in US healthcare is spent on type 2 diabetes, according to the American Diabetes Association.

So, what is type 2 diabetes and how does it work? This disease results from a resistance to insulin within the body. What does this mean in plain English? It means your body either does not produce the insulin it needs or for some reason it is incapable of effectively. Using the insulin it does produce. On the other hand, type 1 diabetes is an autoimmune disease that prevents the body from making any further insulin. Type 1 develops in a matter of weeks. It can take years to develop type 2.

With type 2 the pancreas produces insulin in order for your body to use the sugar or glucose that you put into it. As time goes on the pancreas makes insulin or your cells become resistant to using it. This causes the buildup of sugar in your blood cells and leads to serious concerns such as strokes, heart disease, poor circulation, blindness, kidney failure and even death.

In type 1 diabetes your pancreas doesn't make any insulin at all. Whereas in type 2 are mostly lifestyle factors that influence the production or use of insulin. Type 1 is found in children and young adults whereas most of type 2 is in older adults. Type one is not a disease you can prevent, but type 2 is.

There are significant differences between the two types of diabetes; however, they are both a problem with the hormone insulin. Insulin regulates sugar in the cells and particularly in the blood cells. If you do not have enough effective insulin, sugar will build up in the blood and cause hyperglycemia. This condition of high blood sugar will start to slowly impact the body. Serious hyperglycemia can cause loss of consciousness, coma or even death.

At first you might just feel extra thirsty or experience an increase in having to urinate. As it develops and if untreated, diabetes will eventually cause irreparable damage to nerves, blood vessels and circulation, eyes, heart and kidneys. Living with and managing diabetes of any kind is intensive, time consuming and expensive.

If you have type 2 diabetes and want to control it, you need to eat the right things, exercise and make choices for your health every day. You need to test your blood sugar levels at least a few times a week and eventually a few times a day. You may be prescribed medication to take daily or weekly.

This is especially difficult in the early days after diagnosis if you are under 50 at the time. Let's face it! It is hard for us at age 30-40 when we feel fine to accept the restrictions that come with type 2 diabetes. Let me tell you most of us Boomers with type 2 wish we had started to manage it much sooner than we did.

The exact cause of diabetes is not really known. Yet it is likely that both the environment and genetics are factors. If you have a family history of diabetes then you have a high risk factor. Type 2 diabetes is more prevalent in certain ethnic groups than in others. Native Americans Latinos and African Americans are more likely to acquire Type 2 than other ethnic groups. Your risk is greater if you're over 40.

But no matter your risk, two of the most important factors in the development of type 2 diabetes are obesity and inactivity. These two factors are responsible for almost all of the Type 2 cases in the United States. The insulin resistance found in type 2 is usually attributed to obesity, inactivity and a sedentary lifestyle.

In more than two-thirds of the type 2 diabetes cases the patient admits to their weight negatively impacting their health. The same group admits to rarely exercising. Over 50% of these patients also report sleeping difficulties. Many baby boomers have been living with type 2 for more than a decade. Still many of us don't realize how serious the consequences of this disease can be. Type 2 diabetes requires changes in your lifestyle whether you want to make them or not. You will suddenly find yourself testing your blood sugar many times a day, having more frequent doctor visits, and thinking about diet and exercise in a way you haven't before.

For many of us baby boomers these changes occur when we are diagnosed. For some of us, however, we live with the disease for decades before being concerned about its consequences. We simply don't realize how serious the consequences of this disease can be.

If your type 2 diabetes is well-managed undo oral medication and your A1C results are consistently within range, you may be fooled into believing there are no consequences. This is a mistake and it can be a costly one. Why? Because it allows us to fool ourselves into eating those Big Macs thinking there won't be any consequences. It allows us to fool ourselves into a sedentary lifestyle, thinking we can always fix it later.

However complications from type 2 diabetes occur whether you know they're happening or not. While you think your diabetes is managed, neuropathy is creeping into your system. Little by little your hands and feet begin to feel the results of this. Little by little your circulatory system is shutting down. Little by little your eyes can be affected all while you think you're managing the disease well.

What's the worst case scenario? There are many - yes there's serious risk of heart disease and stroke. However, most of us forget the serious risk of kidney disease as well. Have you ever been to a dialysis center? One look around will tell you the consequences of kidney disease and they're not good. Dialysis will save your life if you have end stage kidney disease but it takes a toll as well. Just take a look around and you'll see a lot of amputees - the consequences of circulatory problems.

Type 2 diabetes is nothing to fool around with. So if you reach retirement age without contracting it, pay attention to the lifestyle issues that can cause it. If you're the youngest of the Baby Boomers and you're either pre-diabetic or not diabetic it's time to give up the Big Macs and Shakes. It's time to hit the gym, to make sure you don't sit in a chair all day. It's worth doing all of these things to keep the specter of diabetes from your door.

Overcoming Type 2 Diabetes

It's not all bad news however; you can overcome type 2 diabetes. You can make lifestyle changes even after you've contracted the disease that will keep you healthy for a long time. There are many success stories of others overcoming the consequences of type 2 and managing the disease well. My point here however, is to be sure that we Baby Boomers understand how serious type 2 diabetes is. Then we can take steps to manage it better. Because if we don't it will cost us financially as well as physically.

So if your doctor tells you you're pre-diabetic all your A1C says you are already diabetic it doesn't have to be the end of the world. Let it be a wake-up call to change your lifestyle and do the things necessary to stay healthy. To many baby boomers this means eating healthier, managing their weight, drinking less alcohol, and being more active.

Some recent surveys show baby boomers feel pretty good about how they're managing the disease. Most of them feel supported by their families. Most of them feel that they know enough to manage it well. Eating a diet low in carbs with moderate protein and low sugar seems to work well for this group of Boomers.

Still even this group reports difficulty maintaining healthy weight. Even this group reports feeling anxious, exhausted, and guilty about how they're managing their diabetes. And stress doesn't help the condition. So if you have type 2 diabetes just be realistic and how you manage it. A plate of pasta every few weeks might not be a bad thing.

Eating spaghetti and meatballs every single night however, is heading in the wrong direction. Don't expect yourself to be perfect but don't live as if you don't have diabetes. A healthy diet and an active lifestyle are the keys to managing this disease, and avoiding its worse consequences. Yes there is plenty of work involved, but the payoff is more than worth it.

I think one of the problems for many Boomers is that payoff is in what doesn't happen, not in what does. It's not a tangible reward you can hold in your hands. It's avoiding the worst consequences of blindness, severe neuropathy, chronic kidney disease, and/or heart disease.

In our instant gratification culture it's much harder to see the reward in what doesn't happen. Managing type 2 diabetes is a full-time job. One in which the payoff is not developing the consequences rather than a tangible reward you can hold in your hands. This can lead to not managing the disease at all, something we baby boomers cannot afford to do. "Diabetes burnout" is something we must avoid. So keep it positive. Yes it's very serious but you can manage it. You can live a healthy life with type 2 diabetes. You can avoid the serious consequences of the disease. With so many baby boomers having type 2, you're certainly not alone in your journey.

Let's review

Type 2 diabetes is very common in the United States. Within all Americans probably one out of every ten has been diagnosed with the disease. However for Bloomers it's one out of every four. Type 2 diabetes is the seventh leading cause of death in the United States. Type 2 diabetes occurs when either your pancreas does not make enough insulin or your body cannot effectively use what it does make.

Major factors contributing to a diagnosis of type 2 diabetes include obesity and an inactive lifestyle. For us Boomers it can also be a very expensive disease. Many seniors find it hard to follow their doctor's orders simply because they can't afford it. It can cost about $10,000 a year for one person's diabetic treatment.

Most of us are already pretty stressed about the cost of insurance and whether our resources will meet our needs. It costs more to eat healthy or go to a gym. We've all noted with concern the increase in cost of insulin on an annual basis. The new were more effective oral medications are also much more expensive and insurance requires that their use be justified.

How many Boomers can afford hundreds of dollars in co-pays for medication? Sometimes there's help available for the co-pays but often your doctor has to prescribe less effective medication that you can afford. The better answer is to control your diabetes through healthy eating and exercise. Doctors need to be brutally honest when they diagnose type 2 diabetes. We need to know the seriousness of the consequences if we don't change our lifestyles. The diagnosis needs to be a wake-up call for lifestyle changes.

One Man's Journey with Type 2 Diabetes

I was born 74 years ago in 1948, the oldest of seven siblings, two who were adopted and my two younger brothers were twins. There are only three of us as of the writing of this book. One of my brothers went missing in action and my sister died of heart disease. The other two boys passed away from Parkinson's disease and from complications of diabetes. My surviving brothers are both currently struggling with diabetes and mobility issues due to obesity. I find myself now battling to stay healthy with both Diabetes and heart disease that both shook my world with my onset of Covid 19. Covid changed everything for me and nearly took my life. Until then my diabetes was controlled with metformin. Not anymore two types of insulin are my refrigerators best friend. I even bought a solar fridge unit I can plug into my truck or camper in an emergency.

My mother was a type 2 diabetic, an alcoholic and a heavy smoker. She passed away many years ago due to complications from diabetes and heart failure. On the other hand, my father had mobility issues from childhood polio but was otherwise in good health. I was his caregiver for five years before he passed away at the ripe old age of 90.

I was a pretty active person growing up. I played college football and was an avid boater off the coast of Catalina in the Pacific Ocean. I love to swim, scuba dive, water ski, and fish. I was 'Captain of mayhem and disorderly conduct'. I was so active I tore the ACL in both knees. This required surgery and a replacement. Then I dislocated my collarbone in a motorcycle accident and suffered from numerous other broken bones.

When I was 21 I joined the army and became a military MP. One of my most vivid memories is escorting Jane Fonda off Fort Ord as she was trespassing while protesting the Vietnam War. After my honorable discharge, I joined the LAPD and Harbor Patrol. After doing that for a while I became a tool and die maker which I enjoyed immensely. I really like working with my hands.

It was during this time, and I was in my mid-fifties, that I was diagnosed with type 2 diabetes. During a routine physical exam it was found that I had protein in my urine which was an indicator for diabetes. I went on Metformin to control it for many years.

I was my dad's caregiver and six months after he passed I moved from California to Arizona. I had no reason to stay in California because both my kids lived in Hawaii. I have been divorced twice and had one child from each marriage.

I was 68 when I decided to retire and go to work for myself as a pilot car driver for the oversized Trucking industry. This was a great retirement job as I worked when I wanted to and got to see a lot of the country at the same time.

It was Christmas December 2020, Lyn and I were eating dinner when I suddenly became very tired, very weak. She luckily a registered nurse knew the signs and rushed me to the hospital. It was covid and I had pneumonia. My heart had gone into Afib and I was touch and go. I was kept in the hospital for seven days. I seriously thought I was knocking at "Heaven's Door". While I was in the hospital Afib had reared its ugly head. The doctors said it was most likely the result of covid. When I was discharged I had to continue to have cardiac appointments, tests, and now meds to control this issue. I was officially feeling like my age had caught up with me.

Covid had really kicked my butt from an avid Harley rider with Lyn to an easy chair for months. Thank God for her saving my life. You see I am stubborn and don't tell me I don't feel good.

Now my diabetes was also out of control which resulted in new prescriptions for long-acting and short-acting Insulin, in addition to the metformin I was already taking. I still use all these medications today. However the good news is I have been able to get off of all the cardiac meds except Metoprolol, for my blood pressure. I had to lose weight and pay attention to what I was putting in my face. Thanks again to Lyn my personal nurse I got it together. I am a big guy like 6'2 and can carry 275 pounds. With diabetes ravaging my legs and feet my career as a professional driver is challenging. I never saw this coming!

Today I'm still working and really enjoy remote camping with my special lady, Lyn and our beautiful German

Shepherd Chloe. During Covid Lyn was a hospice nurse in several nursing homes .It was a very hard job and after my episode she finally retired and enjoys her beautiful yard and pool. Now my biggest issue beside the diabetes is with limitations of flexibility from those torn ACLs I'm very blessed at this time and enjoying life as much as we can. I just wish I had taken better care of myself when I was young. What were we told by our parents? Hindsight is 20/20.

From Maggie

My *Sugar Sick* Story

After a lifetime of eating junk food now my body is sick. Once I eat a piece of candy my body reacts like I never knew that it could. The sensations go to my nerves and my bones start to ache. I get headaches and dizzy spells. Even though I have to watch what I eat, sugar is silent and sometimes it creeps up and down every day. I never know but I can just feel the sugar withdrawal, sleeping every chance I get, meds making me lose weight, little portions on my plate, sweating sugar out my pores, I'm so sick I can't take it anymore.

Copyright © Marzellia Blue

This is just a postscript that I found which really describes several of my Boomer friends. I am not a sugar freak anymore and try to avoid it at all cost. The symptoms of type two and the heart disease that tags along with it make all these yummy goodies pure poison to some of us.

When we were kids growing up in the woods of Northern Wisconsin my Aunt Esther baked all week long to bring up a huge supply of goodies for the weekend at the cottage. She was such a great baker. Oh the 50's in the Harrison Hills. Unfortunately the sugar and obesity killed her husband my Uncle Art at age 58.

He was a big guy, and a wonderful guy who taught us all about the critters in the woods and the birds. He took my sis and I fishing a lot. His death came suddenly after running to the lake in the dark to rescue the naughty neighbor girls from his rowboat. They were in the middle of the lake. They had snuck it out from the dock and lost the oars in the lake. Art didn't swim but he rushed out of bed in the bunkhouse to the Lake. Luckily their Dad got to them and spared Art a dip in the water unable to swim.

After the commotion he and Esther went back to the Bunkhouse to bed and Art had a massive heart attack. That sneaky widow maker struck and Esther lost her wonderful husband. As kids it was devastating to us as well as the entire Hundhausen family.

It wasn't until years later that I was able to realize why and how so many of our family members died so young. The generation before us Boomers had their own set of bad habits that were real killers.

Heart Disease - How Many Types Are There? What Does It Do?

Just what is heart disease? How many types of heart disease are there and what does it do to the body? Why is heart disease such a big killer? Let's face it; heart disease is linked to the aging process. What this means for us is that Baby Boomers are much more likely to have heart disease than our younger counterparts. Today Baby Boomers in their sixties and seventies and the highest prevalence of cardiovascular disease in the country. Everyone in that age group both male and female, 70% have heart disease of some kind. Even those of us who are only in our fifties have high degrees of heart disease but men are more likely to have it than women in this group.

Fortunately there has been a decrease in these numbers in the last few years. This is a sign that Americans are getting more exercise, eating healthier and quitting smoking. As we get older our blood vessels also get older. They become less flexible. They are weaker and blood flow is not as healthy as it used to be. If you add things like high blood pressure, high cholesterol, diabetes, or other illnesses that affect the heart; it's clear why the numbers are the way they are. You can add over weight to this list and increase the risk even more.

A recent study showed that signs of aging might be predictors of heart disease. The older you look the higher your risk may be as well. Surprisingly earlobe creases, receding hairline, yellow fatty deposits around the eyes, and Crown baldness can all be signs of heart disease. In fact if you have these signs your risk of a heart attack goes up by 57% and your overall risk of heart disease goes up by 39%.

According to the author of the study, Anne Tyb jaeger-Hansen, "The visible signs of aging reflect physiological or biological age, not chronological age, and are independent of chronological age." Regardless of any other common risks that the study participants had signs of aging found to be predictors of heart disease and heart attacks consistently. The yellow fatty deposits around the eyes turn out to be the strongest predictor of all.

This doesn't seem to bold well for us baby boomers. There are many types of heart disease and I'll get into that in a minute. First let me say that as Baby Boomers we are susceptible to them all. Yet no matter how old you are it is never too late to change your lifestyle and lower your risk.

So what is heart disease? What are the most common types of heart disease? Any condition that affects the heart is considered to be heart disease. There are several different types. Some affect the heart; some affect the circulatory system and blood vessels. Some are preventable and some genetic.

Types

Heart disease in general is the leading cause of death in the United States according to the Centers for Disease Control and Prevention. Heart disease affects Americans of all ages, all genders, and all ethnic and racial groups. There are several major types of heart disease and then there are many more that are not as common. Many of them can develop as we age. this group would include angina, coronary artery disease, Normal Heart rhythms, blood clots, anemia, deep vein thrombosis, arteriosclerosis, heart valve disease, congestive heart failure, high blood pressure, mini strokes, peripheral vascular disease, and aneurysms just to name a few.

Coronary Artery Disease

Let's look at the most prevalent ones. We will begin with coronary artery disease. This is what most of us think of when we think of heart disease. Is also the most prevalent of all the types of heart disease? Our hearts are very strong muscles, pumping 3000 gallons of blood through our body every single day. The heart itself needs blood in order to function. Blood flows to the heart from the coronary arteries.

What happens in coronary artery disease is that these arteries narrow or become blocked due to arteriosclerosis. Arteriosclerosis is a buildup of cholesterol and fatty deposits in the walls of the arteries, often called plaque. It blocks the blood from flowing freely through the arteries.

This means that the heart doesn't get enough blood. If the heart doesn't get enough blood, its tone and function are affected. The heart can't work properly because it's deprived of oxygen and nutrients. The results of this can be chest pain, medically called angina. If the heart continues to lack oxygen the result is often a heart attack and the heart muscle itself is usually damaged. This is called coronary artery disease because it is the build-up of plaque in the arteries that causes the heart attack.

So what causes coronary artery disease? One thing we do know is that it takes a long time to develop. It can take up to 20 years to create enough blockage to cause a heart attack. Often blood clots can form around the plaque buildup. Clots blocking the blood flow to the heart can cause heart attacks and unstable angina. However clots can also block the blood flow to the brain. This can result in a crisis different from a heart attack with blood clots causing strokes or aneurysms.

Coronary artery disease can have different symptoms in men and women with the primary symptom for both being angina or chest pain. It can also cause pain in the left arm, jaw, shoulder, or back. Other symptoms include shortness of breath, heart palpitations, dizziness, nausea, fatigue or extreme weakness.

Arrhythmia

An arrhythmia is an irregular heartbeat. Your heart may beat too fast too slow too early or simply be irregular. An arrhythmia is an electrical problem within the heart. the signals that tell the heart when and how to beat aren't working.

An arrhythmia doesn't have to be a problem. But if it's highly irregular or if it damages the heart then they can cause severe complications even fatal.

Structural Heart Disease

Structural heart disease occurs when there are actual defects in the structure of the heart. This would include things such as blood vessels, muscles, walls and valves. It is something you live with all your life either being born with it or something that occurs at birth. It can be the result has an infection, a tear, or other incidents that occur at the birth. It's not something we Baby Boomers would worry about unless we already had it.

Heart Failure

The other really serious condition that baby boomers would worry about is heart failure. This occurs when the heart becomes weakened or damaged. The damage is usually caused either by a heart attack or by high blood pressure. There is no cure for heart failure but with the help of medication and some lifestyle changes you can live with it.

Medical Conditions Influencing Heart Disease

There are several medical conditions that influence the development of heart disease. These include:

- Diabetes
- High blood pressure
- High cholesterol
- Sleep apnea

Lifestyle Issues Influencing Heart Disease

- Obesity
- An unhealthy diet
- Sedentary lifestyle
- Overconsumption of alcohol
- Smoking
- Recreational drug use
- Excessive stress
- Hormone replacement therapy for women

The bottom line for Baby Boomers and everyone else is that most heart disease is preventable. Even if you already have heart disease you can reduce your risk for fatal events. Just turn around the lifestyle risks. If you smoke, stop smoking. If you need to lose weight do it. Create a healthier lifestyle including eating and exercise. If you have high blood pressure make sure it's under control. If you have diabetes make sure it's under control. Use alcohol in moderation and try to control stress as much as possible.

80% of cases of strokes and heart disease are preventable. You can control your risk for heart disease. You can make a positive difference in managing your current heart disease. The answer is in a healthy lifestyle, healthy eating and healthy exercise.

A Heart Warning Story

I was about six or seven years old when first introduced to heart disease in my family. My parents received a call in the middle of the night. The caller was telling my mother that her father had died of a massive heart attack in his sleep. He was in his mid-sixties when this happened.

Yes he had lifestyle risks. He was not obese and he didn't have diabetes. But he was a heavy smoker and he drank his share of alcohol. In the midst of those factors, there was a hereditary factor as well.

I was about ten years old the next time heart disease struck our family. We lived in the Midwest but our roots were in New York and New Jersey. My aunt's from New Jersey would come to visit us in the Midwest every summer. She always drove out and she always brought my maternal grandmother with her.

Well, I was 10 years old and she was driving out for the summer. She got three quarters of the way here and drove herself to the hospital. She was having a massive heart attack just like her father. In fact she was having what medical personnel informally call a Widow maker. She should not have survived but she did. However from that point on her life was at risk for heart disease. She too was a smoker, had a high stress nursing job oh, and drank her share of alcohol. She was 65 when she died of congestive heart failure.

Next I learned that my maternal grandmother also had heart disease. She had several heart attacks and congestive heart failure. She was also in her late sixties when she died. At this point in time though, my mother did not show any signs of heart disease. She had less risk because she didn't drink and she didn't smoke. She did however have high blood pressure and high cholesterol.

When I was in my mid-twenties my paternal grandmother died from heart failure. She had trouble with clogged arteries for many years but never had any invasive procedures. See how ever was 85 years old when she passed away from heart disease. My father was 90 when he passed from congestive heart failure.

Shortly after this when my mother was 65 years old, she had 95% blockage in one artery and 65% in the other. She soon had a triple bypass and recovered well. My mother lived for another 25 years until congestive heart failure finally took her at age 90.

Both my parents had diabetes Type 2. Both struggled with high cholesterol and high blood pressure. Yet neither was obese nor did they smoke or drink. On the other hand, our diets were heavy in carbohydrates and fats. Our lifestyles were pretty sedentary. So even though they were not obese, the unhealthy eating and lack of exercise took a toll. So I find myself a 66 year old baby boomer with diabetes, obese, and sedentary. I have five siblings. All of my siblings have experienced some form of heart disease from strokes to blockage to angina. So far I've been pretty lucky. I have no heart disease. I do however have pulmonary arterial hypertension probably caused by sleep apnea, I also have complications from diabetes like neuropathy in my hands and feet and lower kidney numbers.

My commitment now is to stop trying to kill myself with my unhealthy lifestyle and make the changes necessary to be healthy. This means changing my diet, better management of my diabetes, and an ongoing exercise program. With a personal history of diabetes and a family history of heart disease I run the risk of complications from both. However, it's not too late for me. Lifestyle changes can and will be made.

Chapter 4

Storytime: A Type 2 Diabetes Story

Story of Sandy is dandy

To truly understand everything I have been through, it's always better to have some history behind it. I know now, through growing and learning that our mental attitude and outlook in life plays a big part in our everyday health.

I come from a family where most everyone was very obese. The average weight on my mom's side of the family was 400-500 pounds. In my younger years, I was always physically fit and played sports and had a really good build. But family genetics & weight issues have always been a big concern.

My mother was very manipulating and very controlling which I know now contributed to a lot of insecurity and some depression in my childhood years. In late adulthood, I learned that a lot of stress can cause your cortisol levels to increase and can lead to a lot of weight gain, especially in the mid-section. There was an enormous amount of stress due to my parents controlling & abusive behavior, that caused a lot of anxiety. Even with my two younger brothers, this was true. Due to my childhood and genetics, when I hit the age of 40 yrs old, everything kicked in and my health spiraled out of control.

I started having alot of health issues. I was diagnosed with type 2 diabetes. My weight was now 215 and I was miserable. I started getting tumors everywhere, every year it was somewhere different. Brain, breasts, ovaries, tonsils. Each time I was told that the doctors thought I had cancer. I started gaining unexplained weight. My blood pressure was an average of 224/118 (normal is 120/80 so I was at a stroke level). I had severe anemia, and was put on diabetic medications because my A1C was over 8.0 (It needs to be under 5.9-this averages out your blood sugar over a period of 3 months).

I was only eating 800 calories a day and exercising 4-5 days a week. My hands and feet would start itching so bad that I literally wanted to cut them off. They would also break out in large hives and were so swollen I couldn't put on my shoes or XL gloves at the hospital. (I normally wear medium). The pain was so bad that nothing helped and I was becoming more and more depressed. Now reaching a weight of 306 pounds. I felt helpless and everything was out of control, no matter what I did.

I had over 10 surgeries within 12 years. Finally, I'd had enough. Something HAD to be done. Someone needed to figure out what was going on because something certainly was. I also felt that I was genetically screwed up with my health declining and having all these issues. It was not normal for someone of my age and active lifestyle.

So, I started by talking to my primary doctor who did absolutely nothing. I ended up going to another primary care doctor. I explained to him everything I went through and I wanted a physician to work together with me. Together we could find answers and find a solution. He agreed and went full force in ordering tests and going over them with me.

One thing we found out is that my endocrinologist kept saying there was no issue with my thyroid. Well, my primary doctor disagreed and with the additional thyroid studies he did, found that there was indeed an issue. My hormones in my stomach and intestines were talking with my thyroid and causing a huge majority of all these issues.

The only way to help with this was to do bariatric surgery. Still there was only a 90% chance that it would help. It was a risk I was willing to take. But of course I had serious anxiety about having such a surgery. On September 12, 2019 I went through the surgery and my life was about to change forever.

Now I was dealing with healing and learning how to eat again. All this while keeping my job at the hospital. Out of nowhere the Covid pandemic hit the world. I worked at the hospital in phlebotomy and on the front-line during the entire pandemic. The serious landslide of patients and testing began in February 2020.I had lost 60 pounds and was starting to feel way better but my work schedule was overwhelming and my health was again at risk. If I may shed some light on those conditions for a moment...

Most of the country stressed out on how the nurses and doctors had to deal with the pandemic and the conditions. But the lab & the phlebotomists were not getting much coverage in the news media. We were the workhorse of collections of blood and Covid testing of everyone.

Doctors and nurses didn't see everyone. Just those who came to their offices or in ER. The conditions were beyond what any non-medical person can even imagine. I personally worked from 4am-9pm every day because there was not enough staff. Covid hit our staff hard and at one time there were hundreds of workers out due to covid. We all had our shots but still got sick. I was given only 5 days off when I got it because we were so short staffed. We were testing 500 plus patients a day.

Many caregivers quit due to mandatory overtime. Patients became abusive and more aggressive because of the long waits in lines. I had been threatened several times. I was often left to work by myself with no breaks and very long waits. Eating my daily nutrition and then being sick with Covid was not an experience I would want anyone to ever endure.

In all, during 2020 I worked 900 hours in just overtime alone. In 2021, I worked just over 1000 hours in just overtime. No hazard pay, no pay raises, we kept on because we knew how important our jobs were. I was determined to keep my strength and endurance to achieve my health. Learning that my mental health now was more important than ever.

The bariatric procedure is life changing and I have seen too many people not do well, because they go back to bad habits and gain even more. I am so thankful and blessed to announce that I am coming upon 3 years after I had the procedure done. I have lost a total of 140 pounds. I am off my blood pressure and diabetic meds altogether. My average blood pressure is stable below average and my A1C is down to 5.0. My lipids (Cholesterol & triglycerides) used to be over 200 (doctors want them below 150) I have mine down to 73. My good cholesterol (HDL) should be above 45. I was average in the 20's. Now I am at 78.

I eat so much healthier than ever and turned one of my bedrooms into a weight room for exercise. (I decided to do this due to Covid and gyms were closed for months). I no longer have hands and feet that itch, and my anemia is also gone.

It's a fight that I intend to keep fighting. It has rebuilt my self confidence in who I am and how much better I feel and look. I had planned to retire at 65 but honestly after the war that waged with covid and my own health I am working at getting out in a couple years. I will have to find something part time to sustain but need less stress. I only pray we will never experience anything like the pandemic again.

Thank you for taking the time to read my story. I hope this will inspire you to keep on fighting for your health. Obesity and diabetes are a deadly combination. You can do this trust me if I could make it through with my odds so against me you can too. Take Care my friends. Sandy

Chapter 5

Storytime: A Heart Disease Story

Straight From the Heart

I'm 61 years old and I've struggled with obesity all my life. I have high blood pressure and I have diabetes. I also have a strong family history of heart disease. Every fall I get a bout of bronchitis and I have a little bit of asthma. Last year when I began coughing and wheezing I thought it was just my bout of bronchitis. I did have some minor pain in between my shoulder blades, but I didn't think much of it. I had arthritis and I was used to having pain.

So I called my doctor who agreed it was probably our annual bronchitis, and she prescribed Albuterol in a nebulizer, with breathing treatments three or four times a day. She also prescribed an antibiotic. So I proceeded with the treatments I was used to doing every fall. A month later I was feeling even worse. Suddenly I couldn't even breathe well enough to walk down the hall. Before this I had been walking my dog at least three miles a day. Now I couldn't walk 300 ft. something was wrong and it wasn't bronchitis or asthma.

I took a covid test and it was negative. Still, the inability to breathe was getting worse. I had to get friends to walk my dog because I couldn't do it. I was exhausted, yet I had no chest pain, no pain at all other than the arthritis. I simply couldn't breathe. And suddenly I was sweating all over, soaking my clothes, with sweat dripping off my face.

I had an oximeter so I checked my oxygen level. It was 98 to 100%. How could my oxygen level be so good if I couldn't breathe? Was I having a panic attack? Was that all it was? At the same time my heart was racing. But that could be a panic attack as well, couldn't it?

I called my doctor and she urged me to take myself to the Heart Hospital ER. So I did so. By the time I walked from my car to the hospital ER entrance I could not breathe. A nurse saw me and came running with a wheelchair. Still I had no pain. I had no pressure on the chest. However I was a little nauseous. Of course in the ER they ran all the usual blood tests, chests x-rays, CT scans, Etc and yes I had a heart attack.

Now came the questions about family history where heart disease was pretty rampant. My father died of a massive heart attack when I was in my twenties. One of my sisters had a heart attack when she was 33 and bypass surgery when she was 63. A couple of my brothers have had strokes. But I had my heart checked out a few years before and everything was fine. I never considered that my 'bronchitis' might be a heart attack.

While I was in the hospital course they ran all those tests over again and ordered a cardiac catheterization. Because I have had no symptoms and I have no pain I was shocked when the doctor informed me that I had five blockages. One of which was at 95%. Soon I was on my way to open heart surgery.

My recovery was excellent. I went home and within 3 months was able to start cardiac rehabilitation. So it's a year later. I've lost 50 lbs. I exercise every day. I eat healthy, I get rest and I take care of my heart. I'm 66 years old and I'm healthier than I've ever been in my life.

Now don't think I'm saying you should have a heart attack and open heart surgery before you get healthy. No, I'm advocating just the opposite. Start living healthy before this happens to you. It was an overwhelming ordeal and I certainly could have died. If you're overweight, if you have diabetes, if you have a history of heart disease in your family pay attention.

Even if you think its bronchitis, asthma or panic attack, check it out. Find a way to lose weight. Manage your diabetes and remember that heart disease is hereditary. Let's face it we're not spring chickens anymore. We're Baby Boomers who need to take care of ourselves now so we can enjoy our retirement.

This story is from a good friend of mine and of course she is right about taking care of ourselves. My question is as young adults and parents raising our children and working our jobs were there always time? Even now as retiring boomers what is the magic that conquers out genetic malady's? What could we have done differently?

For those of us that have maintained physical body health to keep walking and keep moving, my hat's off to you. You will live a long life and be able to master your health. You have the key to success. Losing that extra weight just 5 pounds at a time will be a game changer for you. Don't be frustrated that it isn't happening overnight. Sandy had to go the real extra mile and take off those 140 pounds. Be patient with yourself you are your best friend here you are living for yourself.

This is my Maggie take on our lives now as we grow older, I am sad that so many of us have gotten to this point of retirement time and whoops we aren't in our best of health. Now a lot of us are scrambling to master that darn Type 2 and worst of worst we have a bad ticker. I am a member of that club. As I write this book I am being scheduled for an Echo and a nuclear stress test again. This time probably valve troubles. I just got settled in to my Arizona casita and here we go again. I won't give up just keep on top of this. Just don't ignore your body's hints my friends, we are too young to die. This is my Mastering your heart disease advice.

Chapter 6

Covid 19 and the Added Risk

The Impact of Type 2 Diabetes, Obesity and Heart Disease on Covid-19 Patients.

The Risk for Contracting Covid-19 if you have Heart Disease, Obesity or Diabetes

If you have diabetes or heart disease the words covid-19 might strike fear into your heart. The risks and the consequences of contracting covid-19 are much greater and much worse for people with diabetes or heart disease. At the same time your risk for acquiring covid-19 goes up substantially if you have type 2 diabetes or heart disease.

Why should this be? Inflammation seems to be the culprit. In both type 2 diabetes and most forms of heart disease inflammation is a major factor. Our bodies tend to use our immune response and inflammation to fight off diseases, viruses and such. At the same time our immune system and inflammation can seriously damage our own organs and bodily systems. When autopsies are done on covid-19 patients, inflammation is a common finding.

Add to this the risk of obesity and you increase your chances of contracting covid-19 significantly. Obese individuals with covid-19, end up with a lot more acute heart failure, myocardial infarction, acute myocarditis. Or a new case of atrial fibrillation. This study showed that patients with diabetes ended up with the worst case of cardiovascular outcomes from covid-19. At the same time covid-19 definitely increases the risk for heart failure. So there is speculation that since diabetics already are at high risk for heart failure, there may be a direct correlation between covid-19 heart failure and diabetes.

However, there is not yet any direct data to support this theory. It does appear that the one thing that is common to all three of these diseases is the presence of inflammation. When someone with diabetes and heart failure contracts covid-19 the level of inflammation increases even more as covid-19 releases pro-inflammatory elements into the system.

Another Factor common to all three of these conditions is the presence of obesity. Obesity is a major risk factor for diabetes, heart disease, and covid-19. Those who already have type 2 diabetes or heart disease are more susceptible to contracting covid-19; it is also true that they are more likely to have major complications from it. These complications can come in the form of an increase in heart disease, or complications from diabetes. Rates of hospitalization and mortality are also substantially higher. If you have both diabetes and heart failure your mortality risk is incredibly high.

There Is an Increased Risk of Heart Failure in Patients With Diabetes Who Contract COVID-19

There is plenty of evidence that if you have diabetes and you get covid-19 it is likely to cause heart failure. Of course if you have heart failure and Diabetes together then your outcome is potentially even more serious. Recent Studies have shown that patients in ICU or with serious cases of covid-19 are two to three times more likely to have either heart disease or diabetes.

Other studies have shown that patients who have diabetes when they're admitted to the hospital with CovId 19 are susceptible to Contracting heart disease.

Given this you can see why persons with diabetes or heart failure are at such risk when they can contract Covid-19. The risks from inflammation and obesity are two to three times higher in someone who has diabetes and or heart disease. Complications for these patients include increased hospitalization and more critical care issues. Morbidity is also higher.

Let's face it baby boomers that means many of us are facing much higher risks in contacting covid-19. Other studies are showing that if you don't have heart disease or diabetes covid-19 can be a trigger for new cases. Then we also have to worry about 'Long Covid'. This can consist of symptoms that last a long time such as fatigue and shortness of breath or it could be something that shows up later like blood clots or mysterious symptoms. There is some thought that long covid might be a form of post sepsis syndrome. Whatever it is, it can be confusing and debilitating.

So your best bet if it isn't too late already is to avoid both Diabetes Type 2 and heart disease. You can avoid Covid-19 as well. And if you do happen to contract one or more of these diseases you can still turn it around with healthy living. We've already discussed the high number of type 2 diabetics on Baby Boomers and with 50% of the entire American population being diabetic the risks are astronomical. Three out of every four Americans are overweight, many obese.

It's definitely time if you haven't already baby boomers to turn your life around. It's time for healthy living: reasonable exercise and a reasonable diet. If you smoke, stop now. As far as covid-19 is concerned all baby boomers should get all four booster shots. It doesn't mean you'll never get covid-19 but it does mean you will avoid the worst consequences of the virus. Wear a mask, keep your distance, and wash your hands. It's up to you to protect yourself and those you love. I am a believer that the choice of vac or no vacs is a personal choice which we should have but I believe I survived covid because I had my first shot just two weeks prior.

For days I stayed home sick as could be with the pneumonia not thinking I could really have covid. I received a call from my Dr's office just checking on me and my shot status and when I told her what my oxygen level was she just freaked out. Maggie you have to go to the hospital now. We will call ahead for you. I drove myself. It took 12 hours to get a bed for me in the covid unit. I was told to make my calls and say my goodbyes. WTF!!

I spent days on my belly getting all the right care and I lived thanks to an excellent team of nurses and the man up above. He didn't want another author up there at that time. My advice doesn't wait to get help.

So let's review. Those with heart disease might be more likely to develop severe covid-19 symptoms. Some of the symptoms might include: Congenital heart disease, cardiomyopathy, coronary artery disease, all heart failure.

Baby Bloomers who are type 2 diabetics also have greater risk of consequences from covid-19. If you're diabetic and you don't have heart disease covid-19 can give it to you. At the same time the consequences and end results of 'long covid' are not really known to anyone yet.

Even with all of this to consider, healthy living is the answer. Healthy living can help prevent the worst consequences of covid-19. And what is healthy living for us baby boomers? A better diet, a lot more exercise, no smoking and lay off the heavy alcohol. Wine is fine as they say. Find a lifestyle that offers less stress and more good sleep habits. Don't avoid getting your flu shots, shingles, whooping cough and covid. It's certainly not too late to get started and many of our fellow Boomers have already done so. If you haven't, let's face it you're playing with fire. Let's get going Boomers!!! We have a lot of life left to live!

A Covid Story

This is a true story

Marianne was 17 years old and a senior in high school. She woke up one morning and found that she couldn't smell. As with many of us living in the covid era, she knew what it meant. A quick at home test confirmed she had Covid 19. She soon lost her sense of taste, was exhausted and also experienced some shortness of breath.

Marianne was able to beat the virus in a couple of weeks. She regained her sense of smell and taste. Yet the excessive fatigue and shortness of breath remained. Still, she was a senior in high school and anxious to get on with her life. She played on the volleyball team and the basketball team.

A day after returning to school she was in basketball practice when suddenly she experienced a sharp pain in her chest. It was so strong it brought her to her knees. Her coaches were concerned and notified her parents immediately. Since the pain was gone, her parents waited till the next day to take her to the doctor.

After hearing her story and running some blood tests, her doctor recommended an immediate heart stress test. Everything seemed fine. All the tests were negative. Yet over the course of the next several weeks Marianne felt worse and worse. Fatigue was her greatest complaint, but an occasional chest pain came along with it.

Again in basketball practice, she began to have a severe headache. She warned her coaches that she thought she would pass out and then she did. Again her parents took her to the hospital and this time she was admitted. Still, the doctors were stumped and could not find out what was going on.

Finally they decided that Marianne was suffering from postural orthostatic tachycardia syndrome, or POTS. POTS are an autonomic nervous system disorder. This disorder can cause changes in the heart rate, dramatic increases even. It can cause fatigue, changes in blood pressure, and headaches. It is now considered to be a condition associated with long covid.

It is believed that it is triggered by Covid 19. With time Marianne got worse instead of better. She couldn't go to school and had to go back to remote learning, because she was passing out as many as 30 times a day. Her senior year in high school, along with her playing on the volleyball and basketball teams, was over.

There didn't seem to be any trigger for her passing out. It could happen at any time and under any circumstances. Next she lost the ability to walk. She was suffering from a functional neurological disorder. No one knew if or when the condition might repair itself. The doctors were at a loss for something to do to make it better.

This is one long covid story that does have a happy ending. After 6 months in a wheelchair and following a protocol developed for her by her cardiologist, Marianne was able to get back on her feet and walk. She finished high school remotely and despite missing her final season won a basketball scholarship for college. She was well enough to be able to play on the basketball team her freshman year. Because Marianne was a fighter and because she reacted to her symptoms immediately, no one gave up on her. She was able to overcome the consequences of long covid and live a normal life.

This lovely young woman mastered her heart disease at a very tender age. Her story is a staunch reminder to us senior warriors that we all should have the will to go on to fight on and do what it takes to make this time of our lives matter the most.

Chapter 7

Covid and the Cost of Healthcare in Retirement

The Costs of Healthcare for these diseases: Type 2 Diabetes and Heart Disease

Cost of Covid on the Health Care System

This will be a short chapter on the costs of healthcare in retirement, especially if you have heart or diabetic issues. These costs are now influenced by the impact of Covid 19 on the healthcare system. Shortages of equipment and people have been part of this result along with the expected financial costs. All of these costs get passed on to us. So can we afford to retire at all or must we work until we are too sick to do anything at all?

The Costs of Healthcare for these diseases: Type 2 Diabetes and Heart Disease

Before Covid these diseases were expensive enough. Just consider this: As early as 2019 the healthcare costs for heart disease and strokes exceeded $316.6 billion. These costs included lost productivity and healthcare costs.

Following a heart attack, congestive heart failure or a stroke there are emergency health care costs and long term costs. After a heart attack or congestive heart failure, we might experience physical weakness, severe fatigue and often depression. On the other hand, life after a stroke can vary from very little damage to coma, paralysis, memory losses, depression, manic behavior and difficulty in speaking and communicating.

Statistics from 2019 tell us that well over one and one half million Americans have heart attacks and strokes every year. This does not include the number suffering from congestive heart failure and other chronic heart diseases. At that time, this meant that there were more heart attacks and strokes that killed Americans as the combined death totals from accidents, cancer and lower respiratory diseases. Over one million people die from some form of heart disease every year and almost a fourth of these are over 65 years of age. Nothing takes the lives of more Americans than heart disease and strokes.

However Type 2 Diabetes is one major cause of heart disease and strokes due to high blood pressure and high blood sugar. Costs were high enough prior to Covid 19, but the increased risk diabetes poses increases the overall cost of healthcare for Covid.

Prior to Covid, approximately 37 million Americans had Type 2 diabetes with its many associated outcomes and costs. Almost another hundred million were prediabetic. The costs of Type 2 diabetes includes the cost for all the serious complications that can develop over the years. We've already talked about all of these complications including kidney failure, dialysis, blindness, and of course heart disease.

Before the pandemic the total cost for all of these complications and other diabetes diagnosis was over $330 billion between lost productivity and medical costs. But most of all is the human cost in suffering and loss. With these pre Covid numbers the individual with Type 2 diabetes will average around $17,000 a year. Usually folks with diabetes in general average more than 2.5 times the medical expenditures than those without it.

https://www.cdc.gov/chronicdisease/about/costs/index.ht
m

The most common treatment for Type 2 diabetes is Metformin. For those with insurance, Metformin usually costs about $25-50 per month. Those without insurance could pay up to $200 a month for the same medication. On the other hand the newer generation of drugs may be more effective but many can't afford the copays even with insurance. These can cost over $500 a month without insurance. And these are all the folks who are not taking insulin, using an insulin pump or any of the new technologies.

Thankfully, the federal government just capped the price of insulin for Medicare patients at $35 a dose. An insulin pump without insurance can cost up to $7000. If you have insurance your copay could be as much as half the cost of the pump.

After Covid

What was the cost of Covid? Well all the numbers are not in yet but we do know a lot. There are costs that are now built into the healthcare system. There are shortages among staff at all levels. There are shortages of medical equipment. Items like ventilators got all the publicity but more people are on dialysis and more equipment and trained staff is needed. Covid causes more heart disease and all the costs associated with that.

Is there a direct correlation between Covid, heart disease and diabetes? As I mentioned previously there is not yet any direct data to support this theory. It does appear that the one thing that is common to all three of these diseases is the presence of inflammation. When someone with diabetes and heart failure contracts covid-19 the level of inflammation increases even more as Covid-19 releases pro-inflammatory elements into the system.

It may seem like it is all bad news but it is not. It is NOT TOO LATE to change your lifestyle. Exercise. Eat healthy. Stop smoking. Lose weight. All of these things are possible no matter what your age. Many people have done it and you can too. We're Baby Boomers and we will not be denied if we put our minds and hearts into it. Years ago we took to the streets to save other people's lives. Now it's time to take to the gym and save our own lives.

Chapter 8

Baby Boomers - We are the World -

Preparing the Way for the next generations of retirees. Conventional medicine, holistic medicine, homeopathic remedies, planning ahead.

As Baby Boomers we have always led the way and we have changed the culture in every phase of our lives. Retirement is no different. We want a healthy retirement. Type 2 diabetes and heart disease can not only stand in our way, they can end it all for us. It doesn't have to be that way and throughout our lives, we have developed alternatives to the established medical practices. This includes homeopathic and holistic practices. Let's look at a few.

Homeopathic remedies are "holistic" and do more than just treat the physical symptoms or causes of a condition. It impacts the whole person, body and mind, personality and any psychophysiological issues. In addition to herbal remedies, it stresses mental and physical relaxation, exercise and a balanced diet. Homeopathic treatments can actually change your physical wellbeing if you stick with it. You also need to find and work with a homeopathic physician. Many D.O.'s fall into this category and an increasing number of M.D.'s are also practicing homeopathic medicine.

Alternatives for Treating Heart Disease

Congestive heart failure: Some homeopathic medications include Carduus marianus, Aurum metalicum 30, Laurocerasus, Digitalis purpurea 3x, and Naja trip. You might consider vitamin D, Co-Q10, aloe vera, grapefruit juice and Ginkgo. Fish oil or PUFA Omega 3 polyunsaturated fatty acids show strong evidence in research studies as a benefit if you have CHF>

https://www.lybrate.com/topic/how-homeopathy-helps-manage-heart-disorders/eddb26ecffb4ef6530739729201fb106udian.

Heart Attack: Stress, obesity, diabetes, cholesterol are all causes for heart attacks. Some homeopathic medications for these include Arnica, Aconite, Nux Vomica, and Arsenicum.

Cardiac Insufficiency: *Cralonin*, a homeopathic combination product, containing the homeopathic *Crataegus oxycantha*, *Spigelia anthelmia* and *Kalium carbonicum.*

https://www.omicsonline.org/open-access/heart-health-and-homeopathy-2167-1206.1000135.php?aid=19126

There are other alternative treatments for heart disease. These might include what is known as a 28 day artery cleanse to clear arteries and reduce cholesterol without surgery. This is an ancient Greek remedy, rediscovered by a physician after his best friend died suddenly from a heart attack. As so many of us have heard in recent years, inflammation is the victim in most chronic diseases. It certainly is with heart disease. Combat it with the herbal medications listed above or acupuncture. Try yoga, Tai Chi and meditation to reduce stress and lower blood pressure. All of these alternative treatments will work and are safe under the eye of a holistic physician. As previously stated, Doctors of Osteopathy, more commonly known as an D.O. rather than an M.D. (Medical Doctors) are often more open to this.

https://newsroom.heart.org/news/some-benefits-potential-risks-with-alternative-medicines-for-heart-failure#:~:text=potential%20for%20harm.-,%E2%80%9C,as%20yoga%20and%20tai%2Dchi.

Alternatives for Treating Type 2 Diabetes

Joe Barton Offers an alternative Type 2 diabetes treatment kit much like his heart kit. It contains articles, samples, and much information about how to beat Type 2 diabetes and keep the wolves of this chronic disease at bay.

Food sensitivity training is being used more each day to help the Type 2 diabetic create their own personalized food protocol to contain the complications of Type 2 diabetes. Other programs like Copilot IQ use nurses and medical calls to keep you on track and accountable for caring for your diabetes. This program provides diabetic tracking supplies and lifestyle and nutrition assistance. This assistance is based on your specific profile and is personalized for you. Both Medicare and Medicaid will pay for this type of program.

Dr. Holly Lucille is a new type of alternative/holistic physician. She is a N.D. or Naturopathic Doctor. She has studied diabetes and elevated sugar levels for much of her career. She recommends eggs of all things for diabetics. Eggs have a bad rap for high cholesterol but they can actually be beneficial to diabetics. "But new research has revealed something remarkable. As we get older, a crucial *metabolism activator* gets shut OFF," Dr. Lucille says "As a result, the sugar we consume stays swimming in our blood instead of getting used by our cells for energy. Worse still, much of that extra glucose gets converted to fat."

Luckily there are foods other than having to eat dozens of eggs that will turn this mechanism back on. Dr. Lucille has been researching these foods and has identified at least 5 that are very beneficial to diabetics.

- Bitter Melon
- Licorice Root
- Berries
- Nuts
- Leafy Greens

Here are a few more. Apple Cider Vinegar: Reduces the glycemic load of consumed carbohydrates.

Fiber and Barley: Eating fiber decreases insulin concentrations and decreases blood tissues.

Chromium: Without this glucose is impaired.

Zinc: Lowers A1C and blood sugar.

https://naturallylowerglucose.com/adv9comp?utm_source =google_sem_g&utm_medium=cpc&utm_campaign=blood _sem_g_general&offid=blood&offerurlid=blood_sem_g_ge neral&trid={transaction_id}&affid=google_sem_g&affsub=6 44667313160&affsub2=sem_g&gclid=Cj0KCQiAgaGgBhC8A RIsAAAyLfGyISd5j8EsqdVwHzpzVLooeddAZ6HvDPjJzHPdjy1 ZiMG5VhIrOk8aAs4uEALw_wcB

https://www.stamfordhealth.org/healthflash-blog/integrative-medicine/type-2-diabetes-natural-remedies/

Other alternative therapies, like with heart disease include, aromatherapy, yoga and acupuncture. As early as 1997, the ADA or American Diabetes Association estimated that diabetes cost as much as $98 billion dollars in direct medical and indirect disability costs. These alternative therapies can help to reduce these costs.

https://www.ncbi.nlm.nih.gov/pmc/articles/PMC3249697/

Chapter 9

My Final Thoughts

So there is hope, Yes there is hope ,,,always hope…However if we do nothing and society does nothing then the hope we have will either be lost or futile. By 2030 we will as a society be overwhelmed with aging, health-compromised Baby Boomers.

However the cost of caring for the aging Baby Boomers should be much like the cost of raising these same individuals. This only works if we invest in long term care insurance and medical advances; places for us to live and be cared for. There is hope if we integrate aging into the heart of our society. We can do this.

We are the Baby Boomers. We are the Changers. We have been changing the culture and society our entire lives. We can do it again. We will do it the same way we did it before. We will do it as individuals and as a collective. We will individually change the way we eat, the way we exercise and the way we deal with stress. We will individually improve ourselves and in so doing, in great numbers, we will change the collective "we" as well. As I said before bring it on, bring it on. We are the Baby Boomers and we have hope. We are the Hope, seasoned influencers leading the way to our sunset days. Thanks for taking the time to join me on our journey.

Let's Talk

MaggieMastersAuthor@gmail.com

References

https://www.smithsonianmag.com/history/crispy-salty-american-history-fast-food-180972459/

https://en.wikipedia.org/wiki/Fast-food_restaurant#:~:text=Arguably%2C%20the%20first%20fast%2Dfood,with%20outlets%20across%20the%20globe.

https://livinghistoryfarm.org/farminginthe50s/life_16.html

https://pubmed.ncbi.nlm.nih.gov/11455997/

https://www.healthline.com/health-news/less-than-three-percent-of-americans-have-healthy-lifestyle

https://www.getrealaboutdiabetes.com/living-with-diabetes/knowing-your-cardiovascular-risk.html?&utm_source=google&utm_medium=cpc&utm_term=cardiac%20disease&utm_campaign=&utm_content=-mkwid-s_dc-pcrid-597878980271-pkw-cardiac%20disease-pmt-e-&gclid=Cj0KCQiAjbagBhD3ARIsANRrqEvap7BCIE7IPUdNLKBd_UhTimw2yGqG0O6gLZdik_DRN3Th3zrC9pMaAsBwEALw_wcB&gclsrc=aw.ds

https://www.nhsinform.scot/illnesses-and-conditions/heart-and-blood-vessels/conditions/cardiovascular-disease

https://www.mayoclinic.org/diseases-conditions/type-2-diabetes/symptoms-causes/syc-20351193

https://diabetes.org/coronavirus-covid-19/how-coronavirus-impacts-people-with-diabetes#:~:text=A%3A%20People%20with%20diabetes%20are,your%20diabetes%20is%20well%2Dmanaged.

https://www.nature.com/articles/d41586-022-00912-y

https://www.cdc.gov/chronicdisease/about/costs/index.htm

https://www.lybrate.com/topic/how-homeopathy-helps-manage-heart-disorders/eddb26ecffb4ef6530739729201fb106udian.

https://www.omicsonline.org/open-access/heart-health-and-homeopathy-2167-1206.1000135.php?aid=19126

https://newsroom.heart.org/news/some-benefits-potential-risks-with-alternative-medicines-for-heart-failure#:~:text=potential%20for%20harm.-,%E2%80%9C,as%20yoga%20and%20tai%2Dchi.

https://naturallylowerglucose.com/adv9comp?utm_source=google_sem_g&utm_medium=cpc&utm_campaign=blood_sem_g_general&offid=blood&offerurlid=blood_sem_g_general&trid={transaction_id}&affid=google_sem_g&affsub=6

44667313160&affsub2=sem_g&gclid=Cj0KCQiAgaGgBhC8A RIsAAAyLfGyISd5j8EsqdVwHzpzVLooeddAZ6HvDPjJzHPdjy1 ZiMG5VhIrOk8aAs4uEALw_wcB

https://www.stamfordhealth.org/healthflash-blog/integrative-medicine/type-2-diabetes-natural-remedies/

https://www.ncbi.nlm.nih.gov/pmc/articles/PMC3249697/

https://www.mckinsey.com/industries/healthcare/our-insights/the-future-of-us-healthcare-whats-next-for-the-industry-post-covid-19

https://www.healthsystemtracker.org/chart-collection/what-impact-has-the-coronavirus-pandemic-had-on-healthcare-employment/

https://www.google.com/search?q=healthcare+before+an d+after+covid&rlz=1CAUSZT_enUS1041&oq=healthcare+be fore+and+after+c&aqs=chrome.1.69i57j0i512j0i22i30l7j0i3 90.22365j0j4&sourceid=chrome&ie=UTF-8

https://www.rbcwealthmanagement.com/en-us/insights/the-real-cost-of-health-care-in-retirement